Stress Less

10 Balancing Insights on Work and Life

Amy Freeman, Ph.D.

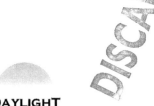

DAYLIGHT
PRESS

Stress Less: 10 Balancing Insights on Work and Life
ISBN: 978-0-9641971-2-1

Copyright © 2014 Amy Freeman

Published by Daylight Press
P.O. Box 333
Bellefonte, PA 16823

Thanks to my sisters,

Wendy and Dawn,

my personal stress management gurus.

Table of Contents

Stress Less

10 Balancing Insights on Work and Life

-A Note From the Author-
The Rest Stop

It's morning. You get up, make breakfast, manage the family or pets, glance at the bills as you run out the door to another job that also demands long hours. All day you are aware that there are not enough hours to complete all the things that are due in the future. At 5 p.m. the engine churns on... social event, grocery store, clean the house, some crisis erupts... Try not to hyperventilate, maybe take a pill. Who do you tell? This was not the plan you had for your life...

While all the problems can't be solved in a day, even a small break from ongoing stress would be welcome. This book is about the creation of small spaces, the rest stop here and there, that allow you to recover and perhaps strategize about changing the path ahead. Take a breath. You are not alone.

Choose Peace.
Choose Change.
Choose You.

Introduction

There are thousands of books about time management, multitasking and doing *more*. This book is about being comfortable with doing *less*, resting and directing action in a way that energizes or brings peace.

Stress is a state of mind as well as a physical condition, both of which are interconnected throughout our lives. While some level of stress is good and serves as an internal warning system, high levels of ongoing stress can be damaging to your health, relationships, productivity and completion of personal goals. This book is for those of us who do so much that there seems to be little time to regroup or plan for the next thing ahead. Success is about finding a healthy balance between stress, productivity, and peace.

The 10 insights provided in this book are based on the following principles:

- You are not alone.
- Small changes can make a big difference.
- Peace and success stem from discovering and following your personal positive truths.

As each of these principles is reviewed further, remember that you are not the only one who feels the stress of being overwhelmed by work and life obligations. In fact, over half of all working people in the U.S. experience this. The business culture is clearly designed to generate income and sustain profits for itself. This means that it is up to you to find creative strategies to lower your stress level in ways that are compatible with your personal lifestyle and beliefs.

> ### *Change something,*
> ### *however small.*

This book is not a quick fix. For most people, it is difficult to take on a large life change or task, especially when stress levels are already high. A more realistic approach is to just start where you are. Change something, however small. You'll find that small consistent changes make a big difference.

It's Not Just You

We are often led to believe that, *It's just me*. But the truth is that it isn't just you. The facts are:

- Extreme workloads are a primary cause of stress.

- Over half of employees say they have a hard time juggling work and life.

- Health care expenditures are nearly 50% greater for workers who report high levels of stress.

- Workers rate the ability to manage work and family as one of the most important aspects they look for in a job.

> **Do your own survey.**
> **See what others say.**

The statistic, "over half," means that one out of two, or every other person you talk to, is likely to be dealing with issues related to high levels of work-life stress. Common expressions of being overwhelmed include:

"I want to run away."
"I want to scream."
"I wanted to stay home today."
"My head is in a pressure cooker."

Ask around. Do your own survey. Ask the question, "How high is your stress level when it comes to balancing your work and your personal life?" On a scale of 1 (extremely low) to 5 (extremely high), see what others say. Be sure to include some of those who don't seem stressed at all. You may be surprised.

Small Changes Matter

Often, it seems as though the "system" or the workplace culture is deliberately set up to exhaust those who operate in it. The truth is that the business system is typically designed to accommodate itself. Any benefit to you is provided with the ultimate goal of increasing the productivity of the company. When considering this, does it make sense to wait for a dysfunctional business culture to adjust itself on your behalf?

The answer is to be proactive in managing your professional choices, your work time and your personal time in a way that supports your personal goals. This can be challenging depending on the nature of your work, its time constraints, and the lifestyle you are trying to achieve. At the end of the day, *change comes from you.*

While it is impossible to change everything around you at once, small consistent changes can make a big difference. A few adjustments in your personal actions and choices can change your stress level significantly, and buy a little time for recovery each day.

Following Your Personal Truths

What we value and believe dictates many of the choices we make. This is particularly problematic when what we personally value conflicts with the values of the western professional working culture. Examples might include differing perceptions regarding the importance of:

- rest
- adequate time to complete tasks well
- time to renew and recharge
- time to develop good personal relationships

- time to enjoy the world around us.

When you understand what motivates *you* towards positive change, it becomes easier to start taking action, even a little. Change is not always easy. *Start where you are.* Begin with a small manageable thing. As you clear the road, the path to less stress will begin to present itself.

Taking Action with this Book

Stress Less includes **10 simple insights** that can help you lower your stress level and achieve a better balance of work and life goals. Each chapter offers opportunities to look at a topic from several points of view.

Several chapters include **short video excerpts** from Dr. Freeman's DVD presentation, *Finding Your Balance in Work and Life: Truths and Myths About Having It All.* These can be accessed by scanning the QR code with a smart phone, at Youtube (Channel: AmyFreeman1000), or at *http://www.amyfreeman.net/the-rest-stop.html* .

Scan the QR code and watch the short video...

After each insight, you are invited to **Take a Rest Stop,** or a pause, to identify one simple place to start at reducing your stress level. If you find the *Rest Stop* exercises helpful you can **download the set** at the end of this book.

Also included are excerpts from the blog, ***Another Perspective...*** *with* *Dr.* *Amy* *Freeman* (www.amyfreeman.net) sharing the author's personal experiences and thoughts about managing stress and change on a daily basis.

For additional information about stress management, feel free to review the list of ***Other Resources*** that can be found online at the end of this book addressing such topics as:

- Understanding and Managing Stress
- Stress and Your Health
- Job Stress
- Managing Family Stress.

Through many of these, you can locate more information on Stress Management.

Start Anywhere!

This book is not intended to add one more major project to your life. Small changes make a big difference. You can try all 10 Insights in order -or just thumb through until you find something that resonates with you. It doesn't matter where you start, just start. Choose something simple and manageable and be consistent. The positive change will begin to spread.

10 *Balancing Insights on Work and Life*

1. *Schedule yourself in first!*

2. *Ask for help.*

3. *Rest.*

4. *Let go of the myths.*

5. *Ask for insight.*

6. *Find solutions unique to you.*

7. *Sometimes, doing a little is OK.*

8. *Personal relationships are long-term investments.*

9. *Take good care of your health.*

10. *Start somewhere!*

Schedule Yourself in First!

Some of the frustration and stress of doing too much stems from the reality that much of what we do is for others, often with little regard for ourselves or our health, both physical and mental. One way to combat this is to schedule yourself in first. Make time each day for YOU, 30 minutes or even a whole hour out of 24!

For many, this is a challenge and flies in the face of the principle of selflessness and giving to others. But- when all of your energy has been depleted, there is less to give to anyone and it is difficult to give your best. You are just as important as all those you assist. Make sure you give back to yourself as well. When you take care of your own needs and maintain your mental health, giving to others is easier and a true joy. You will be in a better position to assist others in achieving their goals without destroying your own.

> ## *Make time each day for You.*

If it's 30 minutes of walking each morning before work or at lunch time, schedule it in. If it's an hour to read a magazine or garden, schedule it in. Perhaps you want to begin to chip away at a large project a little at a time. Maybe a cup of tea and a nap is what you dream about. It is easy to say, *I'll get to it,* or, *I'll be glad when I have time to do this one day...* one day...

Whether it is completing a personal goal or a major project, the event is more likely to happen when it is scheduled in and is a part of your daily routine rather than waiting for the free weekend that may not come as quickly. Schedules ensure that important events are completed. If you are not on your own schedule, this is a message about how much you value your own time, your goals, your personal and professional progress.

Develop a sense of order. Take daily action to keep this order in every area of your life. Creating order takes time. It includes a mindset about how you want your life to work. Detailed schedules and time management won't solve every problem, however, they do reduce the stress of being overwhelmed. These tools will also clearly show you where your energy is going.

Schedules are tools that blatantly tell you how much you are doing. Extreme stress is often related to the over flowing, unrealistic schedule- or it is reflective of too little planning. The calendar and the checklist are but two of many tools that help us in streamlining all the things we do. There are many systems available to organize your life. If you can't find something you need, create it. For example, if you travel extensively, create your personalized packing list. Keep it in the empty suitcase. If you have children, make sure their schedules are included in your schedule. If you are a leader of multiple committees, organizations and groups, identify time to focus on those duties.

If you are not accustomed to writing down everything you do on a time sheet, you might be surprised to find that there aren't enough hours to complete all your responsibilities well. The first impulse is to remove personal time. Resist this urge and think carefully before removing moments of sanity. Are there other things that can go instead?

Get good at saying NO.

Get good at saying NO to events and commitments that would infringe on your scheduled personal time and peace of mind. You're worth it. Treat yourself well.

Take a Rest Stop...
Schedule Yourself in First!

When identifying time for yourself, be specific. For example:

- *I will go walking for 20 minutes per day from 12:00 to 12:20 p.m. for four days a week.*
- *I will garden for 45 minutes per day on Monday, Wednesday and Friday from 7:00 to 7:45 a.m.*

1. **Identify a personal goal you would like to have consistent time for.**

2. **How much time would you need (daily, weekly)?**

3. **Identify a consistent times when you will work on this goal.**

Day							
Time							

4. **Schedule yourself into your calendar first. Schedule other things around your priorities.**

(Download the worksheet at www.amyfreeman.net/the-rest-stop.html)

-Another Perspective-
I Said "Yes" to Me!

I love the holidays, but as November was approaching, I began to see the stress associated with them and my frustration level began to grow. It's not the turkey and holiday candy that gets to me, but all the outside activities that keep my calendar full- in a very exhausting way.

Every self-help book in the world insists that we all have choices. I felt the need to exercise mine. I notice that I have a higher tendency to say "yes" to everyone who approaches me during this time of year. (Oddly, I've convinced myself that I do it in the interest of giving back during the holiday season). So, what will be different?

This season, I think I'll say "yes" to me. What do I want? I want a peaceful, joyous holiday season without the rushed preparation. I want to enjoy the *whole* season, November all the way through to January. I want to feel new and rested when the new year begins.

As I dissected this idea, I began to look at past holiday schedules: business trips, projects due, working up to the minute that the office was finally closed. Some years, I have added more vacation to the Christmas week. This helps, but it doesn't always seem like enough time to recover. (What if I weren't so exhausted in the first place?)

This year, I chose to modify my November-December calendar to reflect only the most important tasks. I removed all the optional events (or re-designated some tasks that were once deemed "important"- over to the newly created "optional" category). Rescheduling is a beautiful thing. I cancelled a long business trip scheduled right before Thanksgiving. I turned down an invitation to an event that included weekend time in December. I cleared my plate for the holiday season I always dreamed of. I replaced late working evenings with the high school Christmas concert. Instead of being in another city, I'll be at my house, deciding on the dessert menus: Thanksgiving, Birthday, Christmas, New Year's Eve, Anniversary, New Year's Day, and all the days in between when cider, wine and cookies taste so good with friends.

I feel better already.

Instead of being in the holiday stress zone, I am creating a place of peace, whether it's in the office quietly catching up on work I've put off, or at home finally laying the new bathroom tiles.

Peace and gratitude are within. I choose to make room for them to flourish. Let the Season of Joy begin!

Ask for Help

In a culture of never-ending work and expectations, it is common to feel overwhelmed and alone. Ask for help. This is the secret weapon of those who manage full schedules well. First, make a list of all the things you are required to complete in a week. Then, identify the things that can only be done by you- and those that can actually be done by others.

Personal tasks that can be shared or completed by others might include: Carpooling for afterschool pick up, meeting a child at the bus stop, grocery shopping for basics each week, simple yard work (cut grass, snow shoveling), having a friend provide care giving for an ill family member for even three or four hours a week or an afternoon.

> *This is the secret weapon of those who manage full schedules well...*

Professional tasks can sometimes be shared by partnering with another group or an individual doing similar work. Perhaps a smaller project could be passed on to someone else who is seeking more experience.

Housekeeping can be a very expensive service to afford, but what if you knew of someone who was willing to do just a few things each week that would make your life more manageable? Perhaps someone could wash dishes once a week, fold laundry, vacuum, cut the lawn. It's not the whole house, but no matter what happens during the week, on Friday, you know the dishes are done- that's one less thing, one less day of rushing, one more hour of peace. Sometimes it's the little things that determine whether you continue or just stop altogether.

You only get help if you ask.

You only get help if you ask. It rarely comes to you by chance. And when you get help, treat people well. Allow for mistakes and the learning curve. When the load is lighter, you have a moment to regain your sanity, enjoy some personal space, or complete the tasks before you without losing yourself.

Take a Rest Stop…
Ask for Help

1. **Identify a task you would like help with.**

2. **Identify people or types of people who could help you.**

3. **Ask three people if they know of anyone who could help you OR**
   Ask three people where you could start looking for help.

   Person   *Suggested Help Resource*

   1. _____   _____

   2. _____   _____

   3. _____   _____

   Other resources:

4. **Try accepting help with this task. What went well?**

5. **What could be changed to improve the situation?**

(Download the worksheet at www.amyfreeman.net/the-rest-stop.html)

-*Another Perspective*-
Cyber Savvy

Some years ago, I set a goal to finally become cyber-savvy. Millions of people with fewer scruples than me are doing it every day. I figured it couldn't be too hard to get the basics. So I set out to learn some new computer skills myself. My goals were to learn to build and manage a basic website, post a photo or video, develop basic social media skills and communicate live across the globe. I wanted to be able to do these few things as well as I can now use the telephone, email or type up a simple Word document. The world waits for no one. I had to catch up.

To the current generation, it is a first language, making them members of a contemporary elite society, Googling this, Facebooking that, checking the web where all the answers of the universe are eternally filed and archived. But for me- it was painstaking. My Facebook account showed everything in the world to all the world. I noticed that other people's pages looked really clean and less busy. Someone posted some very unflattering personal photos of somebody else on my Facebook page and I didn't know how to get the pictures off- so I shut the whole account down! I was trying to learn Dreamweaver, the web developer program where you build from scratch. I learned that it is expensive. I didn't know anyone who knew how to use it well. It seemed to be a specialized skill set. I thought it would be fun to have a cyber product on line, but I didn't know how. I didn't ask because everyone else seemed to understand it and I didn't want to look old. I was afraid to give my credit card information on line (for good reason). I read lots of books and online information- all alone. For months, I was too embarrassed to ask anyone.

The light came on when I saw my 17 year-old nephew on his Facebook page and I asked, *How do you make yours look like that?* He casually showed me how simple it was, set up my new account and told me to call him anytime. He seemed pleased that I was on Facebook. (He didn't call me old for not knowing how to do this. He was one of my first FB "friends.") He explained all the nuances regarding what I see, and what others see, and how Facebook changed their formatting periodically without notice *(so I wasn't imagining these things after all)*. He was genuinely glad to help... All of this was done in less than a very pleasant hour.

That was when I decided two things: 1. Computers are not messengers of the devil. 2. Asking for help is critical for speeding up the process of learning new things and building community with others who support what I am doing. Asking for help invites advice from others and new perspectives. Learning and changing goes faster when you ask for help.

Since that time, I have asked for help to design a website, and learned that there are other tools that don't require me to learn Dreamweaver where I would have to build a site from a blank screen. Several people showed me their favorite systems that are designed to assist the average person in building a website. Most basic services were free or very affordable. Once I tried a few, I chose one that was best for me.

Admittedly, I'm no Bill Gates, but today I can build a simple website and post information to Facebook or Youtube. I now have more than one email account. I finally understand what Twitter is (and rather like the account). I can see why Youtube is what TV was to my generation. I am starting to understand some of the 21st century humor when I watch the occasional funny video with the teenagers. I bought a "smart phone" and I finally realize that the term "phone" is a misnomer- the "smart phone" is actually a very powerful pocket computer that can provide information and communicate with anyone in the world.

Since I began my quest a few years ago, it is clear to me that "this computer thing" is indeed the communication system of the universe. And, because I asked for help and was willing to stumble and try, and re-try, and tolerate interesting commentary of others on my developing skills, today, I can finally hold a contemporary conversation on a basic level. I can speak the language well enough to understand not only what is said, but subtle undertones that have led to new opportunities.

I love the current generation. I still laugh when I think that CEOs of the future will finally make tattoos fashionable for the middle aged. The future is extremely bright. With a little help, I am still keeping up with the world.

Rest

The U.S. takes less vacation than any other industrialized country. This is a symptom of a national culture that suffers from workaholism. Every living thing on the face of the earth rests and recognizes that rest is an integral healthy part of the cycle of life. Trees hibernate for a reason. It enables them to store energy to produce the next season of fruit. Without rest, healthy fruit cannot continue. Only *people* think they don't need rest. Without rest, there is no rejuvenation time for healing and recovery back to one's best condition.

Far more time and money are spent treating stress-related illnesses rather than preventing them. If you have health problems, see your doctor and follow through on your doctor's directions. This might include more sleep, a vacation, or some scheduled downtime from work or other situations that are the origin of extreme stress. Most stressful situations are not viewed as a health hazard, but rather, *it's just my life*. Find moments of rest: a walk, a book, time with a friend, a hobby, time to think- or not. Enjoy some simple pleasure that makes you feel energized or peaceful.

Vacation is just that: to *vacate* or leave the place where you are. If you are in a constant state of motion, vacation could be an environment of quiet and stillness. If you live in constant quiet focus, vacation could be an amusement park or a fast moving trip away with new activities each day. If you are stressed, it is important to create freedom from it on a regular basis, daily, weekly, monthly, and annually. There are many ways to do this. If you are overwhelmed with too many commitments, you might start by saying NO. Others don't seem to have problems saying no to you. Recognize when it is your turn to say NO to others who would add to your long to-do list.

Rest is about making choices you can sleep with. Often we are asked to choose between professional and personal values. Sometimes it is easy to explain why a choice is made. Often, it is not as clear to others why one would make some choices: attending a school play over a business event; taking time to see a longtime friend rather than put in extra hours at work; choosing a weekend of quiet over one that is full of noise and events not valued. Intangible benefits cannot always be measured or explained. Create situations that allow you to choose what brings you peace.

> **Be deliberate about rest.**
> **Plan for it.**

Plan for rest ahead of time. Get your calendar. Scroll to a clear day or week. This might be weeks from now. Mark it off today, with "Out," or Unavailable" or whatever code word you use to reserve hours for yourself. As time goes by, you'll rediscover this empty space at the perfect time. Protect it.

Be deliberate about rest. Schedule it in, plan for it. Incorporate it into your working cycle. What a difference a day makes, and a good night's sleep. Once you rest and take time to reflect, the world looks clearer, life appears more manageable, answers come faster, along with the positive energy to be productive again.

Take a Rest Stop...
Rest

1. *What makes you feel rested?*

2. *Do you feel you get adequate sleep? Why or why not?*

3. *When was your last true restful vacation?*

4. *When is your next restful vacation planned for?*

5. *At times when you are well rested, what do you notice?*

(Download the worksheet at www.amyfreeman.net/the-rest-stop.html)

-Another Perspective-
The Wild Card

There are many games where if you randomly pull the wild card, that card can become whatever you need it to be to help you win that round of the game. And, for a moment, things just work out.

Much of our psychological stress comes from worrying about the unknown. Occasionally, it is important to give yourself permission to allow room for the wild card, the unknown, the chance that good things might happen for no reason at all, that things will work out. This would mean that you don't have to be the general manager of the universe. You don't have to fix everything. It is easy to imagine all the negative things that can happen, but statistically, things could also turn out just fine. Give equal time to imagining that, too. Every now and then, it's OK to just rest and give some situations time to untangle themselves.

Let Go of the Myths

What we believe dictates the direction of our lives. Our beliefs about work and success determine the choices we make. Just as with other areas of our lives, some of the things we are told to believe about success are not always true. Indeed, some philosophies have grown into wildly popular and distorted, closely held myths. Common myths about professional success are:

- *"Thanks to multitasking, more always gets done in less time."*
- *"Life changes can be made when everything else gets done."*
- *"People who manage their jobs well don't experience high levels of stress."*

Let's deconstruct each of these philosophies.

Myth: *"Thanks to multitasking, more always gets done in less time."*

Truth: Multitasking does not always reduce workload stress. The truth is that the system is designed so that you can never finish all of the work. The goal of multitasking is to finally complete that huge pile of work. Sometimes this is an appropriate approach, however, not always. One of the downsides of multitasking is that even though "more" work appears to get done, the quality of work often goes down because less time is available to focus on building strong relationships or think through details of problems that are presented. Also, the more work an employee gets done, the more that is presented to fill in any restful gaps you thought you were creating. The computer was supposed to save us time, and indeed it has made many tasks faster and more efficient. The result, however, is that that the additional time saved is often filled with larger quantities of work to be done.

The mind can only focus on one thing at a time. Contrary to popular belief, it does not focus on several things simultaneously, instead, it quickly jumps from one thing to the next. To have the mind constantly oscillating between multiple events becomes exhausting over a long period of time. Remember, no matter how long the *To Do* list, there are still definite advantages to setting aside time to focus on a single thing and do it thoughtfully and well.

Myth: *"Life changes can be made when everything else gets done."*

Truth: Life goals must be prioritized over other events, or they will never happen. Again, the truth is that more work is created by business demands than can ever possibly be completed. This is the basis of continuing employment. To achieve life goals that are not related to one's immediate professional occupation, it is important to carefully prioritize personal and professional goals strategically. What have you dreamed of? Think creatively about initiating action and taking advantage of opportunities that lead towards fulfilling your personal goals. List the steps, attach a time line, follow through. If later on you are not where you think you should be, adjust your time line and priorities and continue at a pace that you are comfortable with. Do not stop. Do not wait for the approval of others. You determine your future. Make sure that your life includes you!

Myth: *"People who manage their jobs well don't experience high levels of stress."*

Truth: There are several research studies that show that most (50% to 67%) of the working population experiences stress related to work and/or life balance. This is true even when people appear to be managing their jobs well. There is no forum in the working culture to express exhaustion, depression, fear, anger, and the need for rest, peace, health and sanity. This keeps the problems associated with stress well hidden. Keep in mind that 67% is 2 out of 3 people! Even 50% is 1 out of 2 people, suggesting that if you are speaking to another working person, statistically, one of you occasionally suffers from extreme levels of stress. Message: *You are not alone!*

> ***Create personal definitions for success.***

When these and other myths about success are released from the mind, there is room to create positive personal definitions for success. Examples might include:

- I deserve rest and peace in my life.
- I work best when I am under *less* ongoing stress.

- Maintaining outside interests make me more positive and productive at work.

Identify, embrace and follow your own positive personal truths. Actions that follow will often result in the discovery of unique solutions that are specifically designed for you.

Take a Rest Stop...

Let Go of the Myths

1. *Identify a popular professional value that you question.*

2. *What do you actually believe regarding this value?*

3. *What one thing can you do to support what you value and believe about success?*

(Download the worksheet at www.amyfreeman.net/the-rest-stop.html)

-Another Perspective-
Road Signs

Business travel is an interesting thing. For those of us who travel extensively, it is clear that business travel and leisure travel are very different events. The difference is the stress level. An overload of business travel can make you feel like you are forever being pulled away from home and rest. For longer trips, you learn that the world will not wait while you are gone, and unfinished personal projects will freeze where you left them.

Rather than focus on the difficult side of travel, I have elected to see the trip as a part of the bigger picture that brings me closer to my goals, whatever they may be. I choose to bring meaning to each trip I take, looking for a new sign or lesson along the way. Any moment can have a subtext with different levels of meaning among the signs and hidden messages. Of course, sometimes a glass of water is just a glass of water, but the trip definitely becomes more interesting.

The reason for the trip is not always what it appears to be. It could be the business meeting, but it could also be to learn (or to teach) something other than the obvious. This view gives every event potential. On my last trip, the business meetings brought me little new information, but I was able to meet with an old friend where both of us were able to listen, laugh and help each other. In another instance, I was in a long session, getting my second cup of coffee trying to stay focused, and I found that I was sitting next to someone who was new to the business-travel-conferencing arena. I learned that I take much for granted, and that I have been around longer than I care to admit. New people don't carry the historical baggage of those who have been around a while. I learned that I need to make it a point to periodically look at events through fresh eyes and lighten up a bit.

When I returned home, my perception of my surroundings was a little more broad. It was clear that life is not a business trip where all the problems are meant to be resolved by others in a three-day conference. It is an ongoing journey where the solutions come from the most unexpected places, and the answers surprise you.

Ask for Insight

Insight is different than help. Insight is alternative advice or perspective. You are not the first person to have your set of problems, nor will you be the first to creatively solve them. Change is often difficult because we are most comfortable doing what we are used to- even if it isn't the best answer. Asking for insight from others can add a perspective that you didn't have before. The reasons people don't ask for insight include: fear, shame, isolationist thinking (assuming that you are alone in the situation), and fear of losing respect. When asking for insight, thoughtfully choose those you ask.

When seeking insight, seek it from a variety of sources. Consider the success of the individual giving the advice. Was the advice successful when the other person used it? Is the other person currently using the advice? Ask individuals who are like you, as well as those who appear to be less like you. Get information from those who have already lived through this phase of life, ask what they did, what they wish they had done, and why.

> **Seek insight from a variety of sources.**

Often, our views and values about managing stress and work-life balance are generational. "Baby Boomers" tend to work through the stress; "Generation Y" employees are more likely to manage stress by taking more days off. What are the advantages and disadvantages of both? Understanding how others deal with situations similar to your own can lead to creative solutions. Read books about situations similar to your own. If appropriate, ask about and seek out professional counseling or support groups.

Take a Rest Stop...
Ask for Insight

Identify a stressful area of your life. Seek out three carefully selected people or resources that can provide insight about the type of situation you are dealing with. When choosing people, remember that they don't have to be exactly like you. New solutions can come from those who have made different choices.

Resource 1. _____

Suggestion Provided:

Resource 2. _____

Suggestion Provided:

Resource 3. _____

Suggestion Provided:

Once you get insight on alternative ways to cope or manage, don't let fear keep you from trying new solutions. Also, give the new method time to work.

(Download the worksheet at www.amyfreeman.net/the-rest-stop.html)

-Another Perspective-
The View

I went in to work facing mountains of paper and lists of things to do. It was an avalanche waiting to crush me. I sat in a chair, staring straight ahead. I started to work on a small piece of it. It felt like I was trying to fill a canyon with a teaspoon.

I went home to another range of mountains. This time, many were posing as harmless crops and fields to be cultivated for the proverbial greater good or a seemingly worthy cause.   Yet, I could feel myself suffocating, sweating; headache and exhaustion from the thought of it; fear of a new mountain pushing its head up through a volcanic floor. *All of this is killing me,* I thought, *slowly, deliberately, one stressful toxin at a time.*

I needed to move away from the mountains, or move the mountains away from me, or close the admissions window to all new mountain-creating customers.

I asked others if they saw mountains too. *Oh,* they said, *Mountains are everywhere. That's just how the world it is.*

Once I met someone who had actually moved away from the mountains. *It was killing me,* she said, *So I moved. The weather is better. I can breathe. My legs don't hurt from climbing all the time. I can think. I can rest. I can help other people.*

She put an interesting thought in my mind. What if there really are better ways of managing the world than my own? How could I know? How could I possibly change? I am surrounded by people like me. We feed each other fodder that supports the culture of where we are. If I want to change, it might serve me to study and observe those who are where I would like to be, rather than where I am... But I was unsure if I had the courage to learn the path, to leave where I was, to go towards success and peace.

Before I had a full time job, I had many beliefs about what it was and what it could do. Once I had one, I learned things that I didn't know before. Holding a full time job successfully requires a blind discipline to be present, to perform consistently, to negotiate working relationships well, to prioritize the job over many other opportunities, to manage earnings well, to manage my health and family well. Otherwise, I could lose my job. A great full time job is not just a destination, it is ongoing maintenance.

What is entailed in maintaining one's peace and managing stress well? I see the signs. I hear the voices of those further down the road. *You can get here*, they say. *Start walking. Travel light. Find reasons to love the journey.*

I decided to lighten my load, one brick at a time. I feel myself changing directions. The view is getting better.

Find Solutions Unique to You

When looking for solutions to alleviate situations of extreme stress, it is easy to think that there is no answer for you just because conventional answers don't work.

For many, it is hard to find a model that mirrors our lives exactly. This is because you are a unique individual and each situation has its own challenges. If conventional solutions don't work for you, create one that is unique for your situation. Decide what the end result is that you are looking for and work towards that goal. If the end result is that you need an hour of down time between getting home from work and starting the evening routine of dinner, or unusual obligations, then start there and think creatively.

Consider a short term change. Take a Stress Break, for a day, a week or a month. Routinely assign a day each week, or a week each month where there are no stressful events scheduled (or very few). You might consider moving common stressful events to other days of the week to create your Stress Break. You decide what is stressful and why, both personally and professionally. Put in something you enjoy that energizes or brings you peace. For many, this is the precious gift of Nothing: No obligations, no expectations, no judgment, no rules about what you should be doing with your time.

Often, when there is time and space to think clearly, when the noise and fog is cleared away, the solution for you will present itself and can be heard. Your solution does not have to look like everyone else's if it assists you.

Voice your concerns about changing to a less stressful situation. Then, take action, even if it is just in one small area. Take action.

Be careful about blaming others for your stress level. You can only control yourself.

Try an exercise: Take a look a blank calendar. Put in only what you *want* to do for the month or week. How different does this look from your actual calendar? This can give you an idea of the tasks you might want to modify, get help with, or eliminate for now. It doesn't have to be forever.

When the noise is cleared away, the solution can be heard.

Take a chance and change something you've never changed before. Evaluate which responsibilities are critical to you, and which you could choose to stop doing. Have someone else assist in a few obligations, even if it is just for a small amount of time. Consider resigning from an organizational duty that is adding undue stress to your life. Consider utilizing adjustable hours at work for certain days. When you find an answer that works for you, be consistent and stick with it. Change takes time. Make this new solution a part of your routine.

Take a Rest Stop...
Find Solutions Unique to You

Find a quiet place and brainstorm about a specific stressful situation. Name 5 solutions that could lower your stress level. The more outlandish the better. (For example: Fly the children to the moon for 30 minutes! Put all the office paper in a giant envelope and send it to Antarctica.) Upon completing the list, find one theme that seems to be repeated (such as: needed rest, control, freedom). Use this theme to create a possible solution.

Stressful Situation:

_____

Brainstorming Solutions:

1.

2.

3.

4.

5.

Continuing Theme(s):

Possible solution(s):

(Download the worksheet at www.amyfreeman.net/the-rest-stop.html)

-Another Perspective-
Changing Keys

I've played piano for years and was asked to accompany a special presentation of the church choir. They did songs I know, but they chose to sing them in a different key than I was used to. To those who don't have a musical background, this means that I had to play the same songs I knew- differently. This would allow the choir to sing the song higher or lower, using different tones than they otherwise would. When I started to play, my hands wanted to go where they always go... but the key was different, so I had to think and play differently. I know that I could have easily complained and the group would have obliged and followed me back to the same old sound, however, I had to admit that the key change made the same old song sound fresher and brighter with a new message for a new day.

So, I chose to change. I spent days practicing until it felt seamless. The results were uplifting for all involved: accompanists, singers and the listening audience. I emerged a better musician.

Sometimes we can't change the current situation, but we can change how we do things. A friend once told me that sometimes she would deliberately drive to work a different way. Instead of the highway, she'd leave 10 minutes earlier to drive through the park. Instead of going through town, she would choose a route through a quiet neighborhood. She said it gave her time to think and look at problems from another vantage point.

Change is good. Stress is often aggravated by long term sameness or feelings of being trapped in a given situation or position. Big changes, like earthquakes, don't typically happen all at once but they are often initiated by smaller ones below the surface. Change is an attitude. Change is a choice. Initiate the change you seek. Circumstances may not change right away, but you can.

Sometimes, Doing a Little is OK

Every day, we are driven to do *more*. It is never enough. Every report, assignment, project, organizational position, service to the community and family obligations are undertaken and completed- and still we are all asked to do more. There is no official measure of what is enough. The human mind is designed to do incredible things, yet there is a limit. Consider doing less, or, doing a *few* things well.

Doing less allows time for the mind to recuperate. Often it isn't realized how much one is doing until there is a pause and time to reflect. This is difficult when the working culture demands never-ending movement and activity. On occasion, it is acceptable, even desirable, to do a little rather than a lot; to do *enough* rather than more.

It is often assumed that others will balk at the idea of receiving less from you, but in fact, others might be relieved that their interaction with you or your organization is simplified. This can lower the stress level of those around you.

When it comes to a job, an organization or a family, what is the task requested? What is required to get this completed? *What is enough?* When are the actions taken more than the task requires? *What is too much?* When is it enough? You decide.

We are routinely encouraged to provide more than what is asked. Do less. This statement is not meant to encourage mediocrity, but rather, granting permission to slow down periodically and pace the work to be done.

Take a Rest Stop...
Sometimes, Doing a Little is OK

There is no award for doing more simply for more's sake. What are your values and priorities? Doing *less* allows time to reflect and re-focus your energies on things that matter to you.

1. *Identify a project that is extremely stressful and time consuming.*

2. *Which parts of this task are essential and why?*

3. *Which parts are less essential such that the task can be completed well, but in a simpler form?*

4. *Can any portion of this task be eliminated, delegated, completed in advance, or over a longer period of time?*

(Download the worksheet at www.amyfreeman.net/the-rest-stop.html)

-Another Perspective-
The Power of The Routine

When I think about how I completed my high school diploma or even my scant knowledge of biology, it occurs to me that I didn't acquire it all in a day. It took years of repetition, learning something here, reading something there, a little at a time until I completed the course. I walked to school Monday through Friday, rain or shine. Once I got there, they would teach us one more thing. Whether dull or exciting, Latin root words or frog dissection, at the end of the day, great or small, something was done. Over the fall season, a class was completed and I had a basic knowledge of the English language, or the anatomy of amphibians. After twelve years of this, I received a piece of paper indicating that I had the audacity to finish something, and was probably qualified to go on to finish other things in life.

Today, when I list all the goals I want to accomplish, the list seems long and daunting. But then I remember, some of my best accomplishments were completed in small consistent steps, like a class. I would tell myself, *Every day, at a set time, I do this* – for 30 minutes or maybe an hour if I have it. My first book of poetry was written that way from 5:30 to 7 a.m. daily, for months. Some days were productive, some were full of writer's block and frustration. But then I thought, *If it were a class, I would have to go anyway- or at least be present.* To miss a class required review and catch up later. To miss several classes is to lose track of where I left off before. Consistency was key. Some mornings I would just go to the desk and look at it, sipping coffee...and then, an answer would come out of the blue. This went on for some time until one day- It was done. I had discovered the power of The Routine.

I question that there is a single fix for everything, but often a consistent routine of small things can make a dramatic change in productivity and stress reduction. I have used this to find time for exercise, time with my children, completion of books, proposals, even renovation of the basement library. When those "one day" tasks prove to be too large for such a short time, or the time isn't there in the first place, break it up into small pieces that fit into a simple daily or weekly routine. Follow it religiously. Schedule around it. Don't be too quick to change your routine for others. Over time, you will see progress on your goal. Then one day, you'll be surprised to find- *it's done* (often quicker than you think). That's the power of *The Routine*.

Personal Relationships are
Long-term Investments

Personal relationships are interesting in that you have to develop your own. No one can do it for you. This is true no matter how good the intentions of others are to act on your behalf. True relationship building must include the personal interaction of all those in the relationship. Often, work or career seems to become a living creature of its own and can infringe on time and resources intended for other more valued relationships. This is especially true in occupations involving extensive travel, or time away from home or your community of family and friends.

Correctly identifying the many types of relationships you have is important and can be difficult. This would include differentiating professional acquaintances from working colleagues, personal friends, and family (which has its own subsets of relationship development).

Relationships take time and there are only 24 hours in the day. How much of it is dedicated to maintaining good friendships and interacting with children, spouses, partners, extended family members and the social community? This is one of the things that help to keep us balanced psychologically. Developing good relationships in multiple areas of our lives can shed light on who we are, in ways that having a single category of relationships cannot. Personal relationships also bring out other elements of the personality that may not be expressed at work, but are reflective of the traits that make each of us who we are as individuals.

Professionally we are often pigeon-holed into one persona (the supervisor, the secretary, the person who makes everyone comply with company rules). Professionally, good relationships are often enhanced by third party representation, through letters, preliminary biographies, gifts and products sent on behalf of someone else.

In real life, you have to actually show up. Both *quality* and *quantity* of time are equally important. There is value in just being present. Sometimes just your presence has a quiet background effect that simply tells someone that you're there. You're not invisible, or absent. The term, *quality time,* is often defined as being more interactive, allowing all parties to learn something about who the other is. Both situations should leave those in the relationship with a positive sense of care for the others.

One single interaction or activity is usually not enough to make a life-long determination. People aren't widgets that can always be systematically scheduled or treated the same way. From the Friday night card game, to annual camping trips, to shopping at the flea market with the kids, to daily conversation over morning coffee, interaction varies in each relationship. Personal relationships are long-term investments that yield long-term benefits to all involved.

If a relationship is consistently negative and stressful, it might require additional time, less time or some other changes to make it work. Consider counseling. Counseling can be applied to all parties involved- or just for you, whether the others elect to participate or not. At times, it is appropriate to exit a negative relationship for the short term or permanently.

Decide who is important to you.

Decide who is important to you. Be sure that these individuals are routinely included in your schedule in a good way. This could be daily, monthly or annually, depending on the relationship. For some closer relationships, this will include some time unshared with work and everybody else. Make it clear that you would give up a working obligation for someone you care about. And occasionally, reschedule something and act on it. Be clear about who is important. In a crisis, who are the people who will support you without fail? Who are the people you want to have good life-long relationships with? These are the people who deserve your personal time most.

Take a Rest Stop...
Personal Relationships are
Long Term Investments

1. *Who are the individuals that enrich your life most?*

2. *Do you feel you spend enough time to build good relationships with each of these people?*

3. *For each person or group, identify one thing you do to maintain the relationship.*

4. *Is there one thing you would like to add to enhance the relationship with some of the people listed above?*

(Download the worksheet at www.amyfreeman.net/the-rest-stop.html)

-Another Perspective-
Tree House: The Next Generation

How much of our stressful culture do we pass on to our children? I question that children always do what we say- but they definitely do what we do. I have often seen myself unintentionally following the patterns of my parents. I'm sure that I am passing information on to my own children as well, but I don't know which messages are getting through.

Some years ago, I built a tree house with my son. I did this because I traveled extensively and I wanted him to remember us doing something together. I also did this because I didn't want him to perceive his mom as a mad woman who was forever stressed out, always running to save everyone's world but her own.

At the time, he was about 9 or 10 and I was looking for a project that would engage us both. I have wanted a tree house since I was a girl. As an adult, I secretly bought a book, *Tree Houses You Can Actually Build* (by David and Jeanie Stiles, 1998). The most telling information it revealed was that tree houses are as unique as the trees they are built in and the people who build them. It was full of pictures. I dusted it off and handed the book to my son. He sounded like me 40 years ago. "Mom, these are sooo cool! Can we build one?" I told my husband that we were headed off to the hardware store to get materials. His response was brief: "I had a tree house once. It was a plank balanced on a couple of branches about 20 feet up in a tree that I climbed every day." Back then there were no child safety laws; you just looked down and knew not to slip.

The trip to the building supply store was interesting. In my mind, traditional tree houses were imperfect things that were made of cast off scraps of wood, rope and old hinges, built over an entire childhood. In stark contrast, our 21st century project would be completed over a four-day weekend with power tools and new plywood. When the cashier at the store, found out we were building a tree house, she asked my son, "So who's going to help you build it? Your Dad? To my pleasant surprise, my son said, "No, my Mom- she's an engineer. She can build anything." I didn't know he had so much faith in me. I didn't exactly know what I was doing... I didn't even have a good plan, just pictures in a book and an interesting tree which had given us permission to attach something to it.

The tree house proved to be a group project with my son and the neighbor kids hammering nails and holding things down while I ran the power saw and my husband lifted heavy things. The following week, I heard the neighbor kid say to my kid, "This is a cool tree house. We need to make some rules like, *No girls in the tree house.*" Again, to my pleasant surprise, I heard my son say, "I don't think my Mom would like that very much because- well, girls kind of built the tree house. I think we have to let everybody play in the tree house." As a parent, I thought, *Mission Accomplished.* He understood what community was. This lesson alone was worth all the pain killers I had eaten over past week. My back suddenly felt better.

Childhood provides a small window of time to make a lifetime of impressions. He will be an adult much longer than he was ever a child. And, to some extent, he will become me. This means that if I actually become a more peaceful person, he will absorb some of this. If I just talk about it all the time, hmmm..... things to think about.

Years later, my son was learning to drive and the tree house didn't hold the spell it used to. My husband replaced the rope ladder with a wooden stair so *we* don't break *our* necks climbing up into it. But occasionally, if I'm looking for a quiet place with a great view to sip a cool drink, a lawn chair in the tree house is perfect. Sometimes I look out and see my son, running off to conquer a brand new world. He waves back at me over his shoulder, the future ahead.

Take Good Care of Your Body and Health

You only get one YOU. There are no replacements, stand-ins or substitutes. Taking care of your health determines much about how future goals are accomplished. The problem is that humans don't always know when they are at danger's edge. Stress is a primary contributing factor to many health problems. This is not to say that stress creates health problems, but many health problems otherwise avoided are often exacerbated by stress. Physical problems are the most common indicators of extreme stress. A few of these include:

- sleeplessness
- over or under eating
- stomach pain
- headaches
- back and neck pain
- dizziness.

It is common to think, *If stress were endangering my health, I would know. I've lived this long like this. I'll be fine.*

> **Recognize the signs of extreme stress early.**

Consequently, symptoms are often ignored until a major health crisis is evident. It is important to recognize the signs of extreme stress early. Common psychological responses to stress include:

- wanting to scream
- wanting to run away
- exhibiting violence to coworkers
- feelings of anxiety
- feelings of being in a continued hurry
- being overwhelmed

Maintaining constant control is stressful. To appropriately give up control can also be stressful because it means you must accept an unknown outcome. Decide what is critical for you to manage. Consider letting go of things that are of lesser consequence. When you give up control, this means that you accept the outcome which might not be what you would have done.

Let others do their jobs. This honors the work they do and allows you to do one less thing. If someone else is responsible for that small part of the project, or making dinner on Thursdays, accept it without criticism because you buy your peace of mind. When is it good enough? When is it enough *period*? Save the energy of generating *more* than enough for events of great consequence.

A small amount of stress is healthy and needed, however, continued high levels of stress produces harmful chemicals in the body and can damage your health in ways that take a long time to repair. The most common illnesses and symptoms that are aggravated by stress include:

- diabetes
- heart disease
- excessive weight gain or loss
- excessive smoking, drinking or drug use
- mental illness.

Taking care of your health should be a primary concern, rather than an unfortunate regret in the future. Don't let stress harm your health.

> **You only get**
> **one YOU.**

Simple steps that can improve your health routine and lower your stress level are listed below:

- Exercise consistently.
- Eat well, especially fruits and vegetables.
- Sleep.
- Take good care of your mental and emotional health.
- See your doctor for regular checkups. Follow prescribed instructions.
- Speak up about the cause of your stress.
- Laugh.
- Leave negative environments.
- Surround yourself with positive people and situations.
- Create peaceful settings.

- Develop a strong network of family and friends. Those who do this tend to manage stress better than those choose to manage alone.

Stress levels are historically higher than they have ever been. Health care costs and the number of avoidable medical conditions have also increased. Don't become a statistic. Choose to take care of your physical and mental health by lowering your stress level. Choose to model good stress management skills to those you care about.

Take a Rest Stop...

Take Good Care of Your Body and Health

1. *Name two areas of your physical or mental health that you could improve.*

   a.

   b.

2. *Choose one small thing you can do consistently in each of the areas above.*

   a.

   b.

Write these two things in your schedule or in a place where you will see them every day. Begin to add these changes to your life. If you get off track, don't stop, just continue where you left off.

3. *What positive differences do you see after a week?*

   After a two weeks?
   After three weeks?

4. *After 1 month, what positive differences do you see compared to when you started?*

(Download the worksheet at www.amyfreeman.net/the-rest-stop.html)

-Another Perspective-
One You

You only get one You. While I like to compare my body to a garden, a car, or a well-oiled machine, it's not. The difference is, if I don't take care of my car, I can get another one. If I let my garden go to weeds or find out that the soil is all rocks and salt, I can go and garden somewhere else. But my body? This is all I get. It's more like having one car all your life; only one garden in one place, and the climate that comes with it. There are no new car lots at which to cash in or trade up, no farmer's market to substitute for the tilling and planting you have to do yourself. That's the body.

If I knew that I would never get another car in my life, I would be more conscientious about changing the oil. I would really worry about the paint at the first small sign of rust. I wouldn't throw boxes of books on the leather seats as often just because I think leather is "tough." I would finally build a garage. I wouldn't so readily hand the keys to just any old body. I would get upgrades when I needed them so that the car could keep up with the changing times and road regulations. I would give my car a name and treat it like a living thing because I would understand that my care for it dictates other opportunities in my life.

If I knew that I had only one garden to provide food or beauty in my life, I would finally fix the fence to keep the rabbits out. I would fertilize the soil more often. I would plant flowers as well as food to feed both body and soul. I would weed routinely rather than waiting until they have taken over the world. I would learn more about gardening, and be more thoughtful about what I planted. I would learn what grows best in the soil and climate I have. I would be more cognizant of the fact that "low maintenance" doesn't mean "no maintenance." I would spray the apple tree *before* the bugs got in. I would cultivate its natural beauty. I would deliberately rotate crops to allow certain portions of soil to rest each year so that the garden didn't grow weak and tired of producing endlessly; smiling until its leafy, fruity, viny face hurt; finishing reports, and dragging around the responsibility of feeding the world, heavy as rocks.

I only get one Me. If I don't care enough to eat well, then my arteries will clog up. If I don't exercise and run my motor, it will rust. If I continue to let everyone else dictate my life and chew up all my sprouting peas and carrots, then there will be no food for me, and none to share. If I don't rest and let the engine cool down, and insist on good routine maintenance, then... I only get one Me.

Cultivation of a great garden is deliberate. It may seem that healthy plants grow well on their own, but when you look closely, it becomes clear that they are responding to a very specific set of conditions. Be intentional about maintaining the conditions that produce good physical, mental and spiritual health. Embrace the natural beauty that results. You only get one You.

Start Somewhere!

It is unlikely that one can erase all the stress life presents, but there is room to reduce it. These 10 Insights are only a starting place; they mean nothing if you don't ever take action. Stress is a hidden factor that is often dismissed or accepted as an unchangeable part of life. When extreme stress levels go unchecked for long periods of time, the effects are often very damaging.

> ## *Give yourself permission to change.*

Getting started entails making a first step, establishing a routine, being open to change, and listening to your inner voice. It doesn't matter where you start. Often the most overwhelming problem comes to mind first, but sometimes it is easier to start in a place where you have control. Pick a place: exercise, health, asking for help, rest, organizing one spot. Perhaps it's a smaller part of a large stressful problem. Find tools and resource information that will help you look at the problem from many perspectives. Once you begin to change this area of your life, establish a routine of keeping this area in order.

Consistency is contagious. This is true of negative events such as continuing bad habits, ineffective communication, and disorganization. This is also true of positive choices like enhancing your health, building good relationships and simplifying your list of responsibilities. Use this principle to your advantage. Establish one area where the stress level can be lowered. As your stress level goes down, you will find other areas that can be addressed.

Consistency is contagious.

Give yourself permission to change. Whatever you discover that helps you will probably be something different than you are doing now. Embrace those new changes that might begin as uncomfortable, but clearly make a positive difference in your life.

Much of our work-life stress is based on ongoing (and sometimes undue) acquiescence to the needs and desires of others. Treat yourself as well as you treat those around you. Say yes to YOU.

Take a Rest Stop...
Start Somewhere!

This is similar to Insight 9, but this time, you can choose to start anywhere. Choose one small thing you can do consistently that lowers your personal stress level.

Write this thing in your schedule or in a place where you will be reminded every day. Begin to add this change to your life. If you get off track, don't stop, just continue where you left off.

1. *What positive differences do you see after a week?*

   After a two weeks?

   After three weeks?

2. *After 1 month, what positive differences do you see compared to when you started?*

(Download the worksheet at www.amyfreeman.net/the-rest-stop.html)

-Another Perspective-
Stuck? Do Anything!

Ever have so much to do that you're paralyzed? Just staring straight ahead at the mountain of things awaiting your attention? To do nothing seems like certain death- to do everything at once is impossible... Answer? Do anything! Pick something- a corner, a small 15 minute task, and start. It may not be the big problem that haunts you most, but the load is lighter even if you shake off a few ounces.

Sometimes this is just enough to open the pathway to the next thing, and the next. When I have something big to accomplish, a paper or a project, I always want to clean up the office, or go and garden instead. Occasionally, I'll just go and do that. It wasn't the project I should have been working on- but when I return I feel better, often spending less time completing the project than I would have with other things on my mind. This method doesn't fix everything- but it can help. Don't just sit there. Start anywhere you like- just start.

Download the tools
that were helpful to you!

www.amyfreeman.net/the-rest-stop.html

Take a Rest Stop and download the entire set of worksheet exercises (electronic fillable forms) that you can complete, save or share. Also provided are links to each of the short videos from the first six chapters.

Each of the short Youtube ***videos*** were taken from Dr. Freeman's DVD presentation, *Finding Your Balance in Work and Life: Truths and Myths About Having It All.* The entire 45 minute presentation is available through Amazon or at *www.amyfreeman.net.* It's an excellent resource to share with a group.

With all of these tools, it is easy to create an interactive group where everyone's goal is to *Stress Less!*

Other Resources

All of these links are also available at :
www.amyfreeman.net/stress-management-resources.html

Understanding and Managing Stress

- **Managing Stress- The Basics**
  http://www.healthfinder.gov/HealthTopics/Category/heal th-conditions-and-diseases/heart-health/manage-stress

- **Managing Stress- A Tutorial**
  http://www.nlm.nih.gov/medlineplus/tutorials/managings tress/htm/index.htm

- **Happiness According to Science**
  http://www.mayoclinic.org/how-to-be-happy/ART-20045714

Stress and Your Health

- **Stress and Your Health**
  http://www.womenshealth.gov/publications/our-publications/fact-sheet/stress-your-health.cfm

- **Chronic Stress**
  http://www.mayoclinic.org/stress/ART-20046037

- **Stress and Traumatic Events**
  http://www.cdc.gov/violenceprevention/pub/coping_with_ stress_tips.html

- **Relaxation Techniques**
  http://www.mayoclinic.org/relaxation-technique/ART-20045368

- **Managing Stress with Healthy Habits**
  http://www.heart.org/HEARTORG/GettingHealthy/Stress Management/FightStressWithHealthyHabits/Fight-Stress-with-Healthy-Habits_UCM_307992_Article.jsp

Job Stress

- **Emotional Symptoms of Job Stress**
  http://www.stress.org/workplace-stress/

- **Multitasking and Productivity**
  http://www.mayoclinic.org/how-to-focus/expert-answers/FAQ-20058383

- **Multitasking- Research Summary**
  http://www.npr.org/templates/story/story.php?storyId=9 5256794

- **Employee Stress and Effectiveness (StressPulse Survey)**
  http://www.compsych.com/press-room/press-releases-2012/678-october-29-2012

Managing Family Stress

- **Building Resilience in Children**
  http://www.apa.org/helpcenter/resilience.aspx

- **Decreasing Family Stress**
  http://www.webmd.com/parenting/raising-fit-kids/mood/slideshow-decrease-family-stress

- **Caregiver Survival Tips**
  http://www.aoa.gov/AoARoot/Press_Room/Products_Materials/fact/pdf/AoA_HealthyLivingTips_Caregiver_Survival%20Tips.pdf

Other Publications
by Amy Freeman, Ph.D.

Self Help:

Stress Less: 10 Balancing Insights on Work and Life (2014)

Finding Your Balance in Work and Life: Truths and Myths about Having It All (2013- DVD Presentation)

Poetry:

A Collection of Paper Ducks: A Book About Becoming (1993)

Cache: A Book About Leaving and Finding the Way Home (1993)

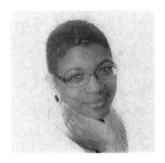

Amy Freeman holds a Ph.D. in Workforce Education. She is also an engineer, an educator, and a working parent who understands the challenges of interweaving family obligations with professional expectations. She has spoken at numerous business and professional venues in the U.S. and abroad. As an advocate of education, she emphasizes the need to share ideas, collaborate and learn as much as possible about others and the world around us. Learn more online at *amyfreeman.net.*

CPSIA information can be obtained at www.ICGtesting.com
Printed in the USA
LVOW11s1601050814

397636LV00002B/330/P